HOW TO RECOVER FROM INJURIES

The Complete Guide to Injury Rehabilitation, Physical Therapy and Recovery Exercises

Robert Monteleone

Copyright © 2024 by Curtis Wood

*All rights reserved.
No part of this work may be reproduced, distributed, or transmitted in any form or by any means, including photocopying, recording, or other electronic or mechanical methods, without the prior written permission of the copyright holder, except in the case of brief quotations embodied in critical reviews and certain other noncommercial uses permitted by copyright law.*

Table of content

Introduction	4
Chapter 1: Understanding Common Injuries	8
Chapter 2: The Phases of Healing	15
Chapter 3: Immediate Response to Injury	21
Chapter 4: The Role of Medical Professionals	28
Chapter 5: Setting Realistic Recovery Goals	36
Chapter 6: Importance of Rest and Recovery	43
Chapter 7: Nutrition for Healing	51
Chapter 8: Pain Management Techniques	62
Chapter 9: The Benefits of Physical Therapy	71
Chapter 10: Developing a Rehabilitation Plan	81
Chapter 11: Stretching and Flexibility Exercises	88
Chapter 12: Strength Training for Recovery	98
Chapter 13: Cardiovascular Conditioning	108
Chapter 14: Balance and Coordination Exercises	118
Chapter 15: Mental Health and Injury Recovery	129
Chapter 16: Preventing Re-Injury	137
Chapter 17: Adapting Daily Activities	147
Chapter 18: Long-Term Recovery Strategies	155
Chapter 19: Success Stories and Case Studies	163
Conclusion	171

Introduction

Injuries can happen to anyone at any time. Whether you're an athlete, someone who exercises occasionally, or just living your daily life, an unexpected twist, fall, or accident can leave you hurt and frustrated. The pain of an injury is not just physical; it can also affect your emotions and mental health. But there's good news: with the right approach, you can recover from almost any injury and get back to your normal activities stronger than ever.

Recovery from an injury is a journey. It doesn't happen overnight, and it's not always easy. However, understanding the process can make it less scary. This book is here to guide you through every step. From the moment you get injured to the day you are back to your best self, we will give you the knowledge, tools, and support you need to succeed.

The first thing to remember is that recovery takes time. It involves several stages, each with its own challenges and goals. Knowing what to expect can help you stay positive and motivated. We'll start by talking about what to do right after you get injured, which is very important for starting the healing process. This includes steps like resting, using ice, and getting medical help.

Next, we will talk about different types of injuries and how they heal. Every injury is different, and understanding yours can help you make a good recovery plan. We'll cover common injuries like sprains, strains, and broken bones. You'll learn about how the body heals and how you can help it.

Physical therapy is a big part of getting better. It's not just about getting stronger; it's also about getting back your movement, flexibility, and function. We'll look at different physical therapy techniques and exercises that can help you recover.

These exercises are designed to be safe and effective, helping you rebuild your body step by step.

What you eat can also help you get better faster. We'll give you tips on the best foods and supplements to support your recovery, helping your body get the nutrients it needs to repair itself.

Managing pain is often a big concern when you're recovering from an injury. It's important to find ways to handle pain without using too much medication. We'll talk about different pain management strategies, from using ice and heat to trying things like acupuncture and massage.

Your mental health is just as important as your physical health when you're recovering. Injuries can be tough on your mind, leading to feelings of frustration, anxiety, and even depression. We'll give you advice on how to keep a positive mindset, set realistic goals, and stay motivated even when things get tough.

Preventing another injury is crucial. Once you're better, the last thing you want is to get hurt again.

We'll give you tips on how to protect yourself and stay strong so you can enjoy your favorite activities without fear of injury.

Finally, we'll share inspiring success stories from people who have been through similar experiences. These stories will show you that recovery is possible and that you are not alone. You'll also find a list of resources and support networks to help you along the way.

Recovery is a journey that requires patience, effort, and determination. But with the right guidance and support, you can overcome your injury and come out stronger on the other side. This book is your companion on that journey, giving you the information and encouragement you need to succeed. Together, we'll make sure that your road to recovery is as smooth and effective as possible.

Chapter 1: Understanding Common Injuries

Injuries are a part of life. They can happen to anyone, whether you're playing sports, working out, or just going about your daily routine. Understanding common injuries can help you take better care of yourself and recover faster if you do get hurt. In this chapter, we will look at some of the most common injuries, how they happen, and what you can do to heal and prevent them in the future.

Sprains and Strains

Sprains and strains are among the most common injuries. A sprain happens when you stretch or tear a ligament, the tough bands of tissue that connect bones to each other. This often occurs in your ankles, wrists, or knees. A strain, on the other hand, is when you stretch or tear a muscle or tendon, the tissues that connect muscles to bones. This can happen in your back, legs, or arms.

Sprains and strains usually happen because of a sudden movement, like twisting your ankle or lifting something heavy. You might feel pain, swelling, and bruising. The best way to treat these injuries is to rest, ice the area, compress it with a bandage, and elevate it. This is known as the R.I.C.E. method: Rest, Ice, Compression, Elevation.

Fractures

A fracture is a broken bone. Fractures can happen from a fall, a direct blow, or a collision. There are different types of fractures, from a small crack to a complete break. Common signs of a fracture include severe pain, swelling, bruising, and an inability to move the injured part.

If you think you have a fracture, it's important to see a doctor right away. They will take an X-ray to see the extent of the damage. Treatment for a fracture usually involves immobilizing the bone with a cast or splint to allow it to heal. In some cases, surgery may be needed to fix the bone.

Dislocations

A dislocation happens when a bone is forced out of its normal position in a joint. This can happen in your shoulders, elbows, fingers, or knees. Dislocations are very painful and can cause swelling, bruising, and an inability to move the joint.

If you have a dislocation, you should see a doctor immediately. They will need to put the bone back in place, a process called reduction. After that, you may need to wear a splint or sling to keep the joint stable while it heals. Physical therapy can help restore strength and movement to the injured joint.

Tendinitis

Tendinitis is an inflammation of a tendon. It often happens from overuse or repetitive motion. Common areas for tendinitis include the shoulders, elbows, wrists, and knees. You might feel pain, tenderness, and mild swelling.

The best way to treat tendinitis is to rest the affected area and avoid activities that cause pain. Applying ice and taking anti-inflammatory medications can help reduce swelling. Stretching and strengthening exercises can also be beneficial once the pain subsides.

Back Injuries

Back injuries are very common and can range from minor strains to more serious conditions like herniated discs. Back injuries can happen from lifting something heavy, poor posture, or sudden movements. You might feel pain, stiffness, or muscle spasms.

To treat a back injury, it's important to rest and avoid activities that cause pain. Applying heat or ice can help reduce pain and swelling. Physical therapy can also be very helpful in strengthening the muscles around your spine and improving your posture.

Concussions

A concussion is a type of traumatic brain injury that happens when you hit your head or your head is violently shaken. Concussions are common in contact sports like football or soccer, but they can also happen from falls or car accidents. Symptoms of a concussion include headache, dizziness, confusion, nausea, and sensitivity to light or noise.

If you think you have a concussion, it's important to see a doctor right away. Rest is the most important treatment for a concussion. You will need to avoid activities that can make your symptoms worse, including physical activities and tasks that require a lot of concentration.

Overuse Injuries

Overuse injuries happen when you do the same motion over and over again, causing wear and tear on your muscles, tendons, and joints. Common overuse injuries include stress fractures, shin splints, and runner's knee. You might feel pain, swelling, and stiffness.

The best way to treat overuse injuries is to rest and avoid the activity that caused the injury. Ice, compression, and elevation can help reduce swelling. Physical therapy and exercises to strengthen the affected area can also help.

Preventing Injuries

While injuries can happen unexpectedly, there are things you can do to reduce your risk. Always warm up before exercising and cool down afterward. Stretch regularly to keep your muscles flexible. Use proper techniques when lifting, running, or playing sports. Make sure to wear the right gear, like supportive shoes or protective equipment.

Listening to your body is also important. If you feel pain or discomfort, take a break and rest. Pushing through pain can make injuries worse. Staying active and keeping your muscles strong can help prevent injuries, but it's important to balance activity with rest and recovery.

Understanding common injuries and how they happen is the first step in taking care of yourself. With the right knowledge and care, you can heal from injuries and get back to the activities you love.

Chapter 2: The Phases of Healing

Healing from an injury is like going on a journey. Each phase of healing is a step towards getting better and stronger. Understanding these phases can help you know what to expect and how to take care of yourself at each stage. Let's explore the different phases of healing in a way that's easy to understand and will keep you engaged.

Phase 1: Inflammation

The first phase of healing is inflammation. Right after you get injured, your body reacts quickly to protect the affected area. This phase can be uncomfortable, but it's a crucial part of the healing process. Here's what happens:

- Immediate Response: When you get hurt, your body sends extra blood to the injured area. This causes redness, warmth, swelling, and sometimes pain.
- Protecting the Injury: The swelling is your body's way of protecting the injured area from further damage.
- Cleaning Up: White blood cells rush to the site to clean up damaged tissue and prevent infection.

What You Can Do
- Rest: Avoid using the injured area to prevent further damage.
- Ice: Apply ice to reduce swelling and numb the pain.
- Compression: Use an elastic bandage to provide support and reduce swelling.
- Elevation: Keep the injured area raised above your heart level to decrease swelling.

Phase 2: Proliferation

The second phase is proliferation. During this phase, your body starts to rebuild the damaged tissues. This phase usually begins a few days after the injury and can last for several weeks. Here's what happens:

- Cell Growth: New cells start to grow and multiply, creating new tissue.
- Formation of New Blood Vessels: New blood vessels form to supply the healing area with oxygen and nutrients.
- Building Strength: Collagen, a protein that provides strength and structure, begins to form.

What You Can Do
- Gentle Movement: Start gentle movements and exercises as recommended by your healthcare provider to promote healing and prevent stiffness.
- Healthy Diet: Eat a balanced diet rich in vitamins and protein to support tissue repair.

- Stay Hydrated: Drink plenty of water to keep your body functioning well.

Phase 3: Maturation

The third phase is maturation, also known as the remodeling phase. This phase can last for several months or even years, depending on the severity of the injury. During this time, your body strengthens and reorganizes the new tissue to make it as strong and functional as possible. Here's what happens:

- Collagen Remodeling: The new collagen fibers are rearranged and strengthened.
- Scar Tissue Formation: Any scar tissue that formed during the earlier phases is remodeled to blend in with the surrounding tissue.
- Restoration of Function: The injured area gradually returns to its normal function.

What You Can Do

- Continue Exercise: Keep doing the exercises and stretches recommended by your healthcare provider to maintain flexibility and strength.
- Stay Active: Gradually return to your regular activities, but avoid overdoing it to prevent re-injury.
- Monitor Progress: Keep track of your recovery and note any changes or discomfort. Consult your healthcare provider if you have concerns.

The Emotional Side of Healing

Healing isn't just physical; it also involves emotional and mental recovery. Dealing with an injury can be challenging and frustrating. Here are some tips to manage the emotional side of healing:

- Stay Positive: Focus on the progress you're making, even if it seems slow. Celebrate small victories.
- Seek Support: Talk to friends, family, or a support group about your feelings and experiences.

- Set Realistic Goals: Set achievable goals to keep yourself motivated and track your progress.
- Practice Patience: Understand that healing takes time, and it's okay to have ups and downs along the way.

Understanding the phases of healing helps you know what to expect and how to take care of yourself at each stage. The inflammation phase protects and prepares the injured area for healing. The proliferation phase rebuilds and strengthens new tissue. The maturation phase restores function and makes the new tissue stronger. By following the right steps and staying patient, you can support your body through each phase and achieve a full recovery. Remember, healing is a journey, and with the right approach, you can come out stronger on the other side.

Chapter 3: Immediate Response to Injury

When you get injured, the first few moments are crucial. Knowing what to do right away can make a big difference in how well and how quickly you heal. This chapter will guide you through the immediate steps you should take when you get hurt. Acting fast and smart can help reduce pain, prevent further damage, and set the stage for a smooth recovery.

Stay Calm and Assess the Situation
The first thing to do when you get injured is to stay calm. It's natural to feel scared or upset, but taking a deep breath and staying focused can help you think clearly. Assess the situation and determine how serious the injury is. Ask yourself a few questions:

- Can you move the injured part?
- Is there severe pain, swelling, or bruising?
- Is there any bleeding?
- Do you feel dizzy or lightheaded?

Understanding the severity of your injury will help you decide what steps to take next.

Protect the Injured Area

Once you've assessed the injury, it's important to protect the injured area to prevent further damage. Avoid moving the injured part as much as possible. If you have a sprain or strain, try to immobilize the area with a splint or bandage. If you suspect a broken bone, don't try to move it. Keep the injured area open until you can get medical help.

Apply the R.I.C.E. Method

The R.I.C.E. method is a simple and effective way to treat many common injuries right after they happen. R.I.C.E. stands for Rest, Ice, Compression, and Elevation.

Rest: Stop using the injured part immediately. Resting helps prevent further damage and allows your body to start the healing process. If you're playing sports or exercising, stop your activity right away.

Ice: Apply ice to the injured area as soon as possible. Ice helps reduce swelling and numbs the pain. Use an ice pack, a bag of frozen vegetables, or a cold, wet cloth. Apply the ice for 15-20 minutes at a time, and repeat every hour as needed. Make sure to wrap the ice in a cloth to protect your skin from frostbite.

Compression: Use a bandage or wrap to compress the injured area. Compression helps reduce swelling and provides support to the injured part. Be careful not to wrap it too tightly, as this can cut off circulation. If you feel tingling or numbness, loosen the bandage.

Elevation: Elevate the injured part above the level of your heart if possible. Elevation helps reduce swelling by allowing fluids to drain away from the injured area. Use pillows or cushions to keep the injured part raised.

Seek Medical Help if Needed
Some injuries require professional medical attention. If you suspect a serious injury, such as a broken bone, dislocation, or severe sprain, it's important to see a doctor right away. Signs that you should seek medical help include:

- Inability to move the injured part
- Severe pain that doesn't improve with rest and ice
- Significant swelling or bruising
- Visible deformity or unusual appearance of the injured area

- Numbness or loss of feeling
- Heavy bleeding that doesn't stop with pressure

Don't hesitate to call emergency services if you're unsure about the severity of the injury. It's better to be safe and get the help you need.

Manage Pain and Swelling
Pain and swelling are common after an injury. In addition to the R.I.C.E. method, over-the-counter pain relievers like ibuprofen or acetaminophen can help manage pain and reduce inflammation. Always follow the instructions on the label and consult your doctor if you have any questions.

Keep the Injury Clean
If your injury involves a cut or scrape, it's important to keep it clean to prevent infection. Rinse the wound with clean water to remove any dirt or debris. Use a mild soap if needed, but avoid harsh chemicals or alcohol, which can irritate the

wound. After cleaning, cover the wound with a sterile bandage or dressing.

Monitor Your Injury

Keep an eye on your injury over the next few days. Look for signs of improvement, such as reduced pain and swelling. Also, watch for any signs of infection, like increased redness, warmth, or pus. If your injury doesn't improve or if it gets worse, contact your doctor.

Take Care of Yourself

Rest is crucial after an injury. Make sure to give your body the time it needs to heal. Avoid activities that could make the injury worse. Follow your doctor's advice on when it's safe to return to your normal activities.

Eating a healthy diet can also support your recovery. Foods rich in vitamins and minerals, like fruits, vegetables, lean proteins, and whole grains, can help your body repair itself. Stay hydrated by drinking plenty of water.

Stay Positive and Patient
Healing takes time, and it's important to stay positive and patient. It's normal to feel frustrated or impatient but remember that every day brings you closer to recovery. Surround yourself with supportive friends and family who can encourage you and help you stay motivated.

Knowing how to respond immediately to an injury can make a big difference in your recovery. By staying calm, protecting the injured area, and following the R.I.C.E. method, you can reduce pain and swelling and start the healing process. Seek medical help if needed, and take good care of yourself during your recovery. With the right approach, you'll be back on your feet and feeling better soon.

Chapter 4: The Role of Medical Professionals

When you get injured, medical professionals play a key role in your recovery. Their knowledge, skills, and care can make a huge difference in how well and how quickly you heal. This chapter will explore the different types of medical professionals who might help you, what they do, and how they can support you through each stage of your recovery.

Primary Care Doctors

Your primary care doctor is often the first person you see when you get injured. They are trained to treat a wide range of health issues, including injuries. Your primary care doctor can assess your injury, provide initial treatment, and refer you to specialists if needed.

During your visit, your doctor will ask about how the injury happened and examine the injured area. They might order tests like X-rays or MRIs to get a better look at the injury. Based on their findings, they will create a treatment plan for you. This plan may include rest, medication, physical therapy, or other treatments.

Specialists

Sometimes, your injury may require the expertise of a specialist. Specialists are doctors who have extra training in specific areas of medicine. Here are a few types of specialists who might help with your recovery:

- Orthopedic Surgeons: These doctors specialize in bones, joints, muscles, and tendons. They treat fractures, dislocations, and other musculoskeletal injuries. If you need surgery, an orthopedic surgeon will perform the procedure and guide your post-surgery recovery.

- Sports Medicine Doctors: These doctors focus on injuries related to sports and physical activity. They understand the demands of different sports and can help you recover in a way that gets you back to your activities safely.

- Neurologists: If you have a head injury or nerve damage, a neurologist can help. They specialize in the nervous system and can diagnose and treat issues like concussions and nerve injuries.

Physical Therapists

Physical therapists play a crucial role in helping you regain strength, movement, and function after an injury. They are trained to design exercise programs tailored to your specific needs and abilities. Physical therapy usually starts with a thorough assessment of your injury and your current physical condition. Your physical therapist will guide you through exercises that target the injured area and help you recover safely. These exercises can improve your flexibility, strength, and coordination. Physical therapy can also help reduce pain and prevent future injuries by teaching you proper movement techniques.

Occupational Therapists

Occupational therapists help you regain the ability to perform daily activities after an injury. This can include tasks like dressing, cooking, or working. They focus on improving your fine motor skills and adapting your environment to make everyday tasks easier.

For example, if you have a hand injury, an occupational therapist might teach you exercises to strengthen your hand and improve your grip. They might also suggest tools or modifications to help you manage daily activities while you recover.

Nurses

Nurses are an essential part of your medical care team. They provide hands-on care and support throughout your recovery process. Nurses can help with wound care, pain management, and monitoring your overall health. They are often the ones who teach you how to care for your injury at home and answer any questions you have.

Nurses also play a vital role in helping you manage any medications prescribed by your doctor. They can explain how to take your medications properly and monitor for any side effects.

Radiologists

Radiologists are doctors who specialize in interpreting medical images, like X-rays, MRIs, and CT scans. They work behind the scenes to help diagnose your injury. By looking at these images, radiologists can provide detailed information about the extent of your injury, which helps your primary care doctor or specialist develop an effective treatment plan.

Pharmacists

Pharmacists are experts in medications and can be a valuable resource during your recovery. They can explain how your medications work, how to take them correctly, and what side effects to watch for. Pharmacists can also help you manage any other medications you're taking to avoid harmful interactions.

Mental Health Professionals

Injuries can take a toll on your mental health. Feelings of frustration, anxiety, and depression are common during the recovery process. Mental health professionals, such as psychologists and counselors, can help you cope with these feelings.

Talking to a mental health professional can provide you with strategies to manage stress, set realistic goals, and stay motivated during your recovery. They can also offer support and encouragement, helping you stay positive even when the journey gets tough.

The Importance of Teamwork
Recovering from an injury often involves a team of medical professionals working together to provide the best care. Each professional brings their expertise to your recovery plan, ensuring that all aspects of your health are addressed. Communication and collaboration among your care team are essential for a smooth and effective recovery.

Advocating for Yourself
While medical professionals are there to help, it's important to be an active participant in your own care. Don't be afraid to ask questions, express your concerns, and share your goals with your medical team. Understanding your treatment plan and knowing what to expect can help you feel more in control and confident during your recovery.

Medical professionals play a vital role in helping you recover from an injury. From your primary care doctor to specialists, physical therapists, and nurses, each member of your care team is dedicated to supporting your healing process. By working together and staying informed, you can navigate your recovery journey with confidence and get back to doing the things you love.

Chapter 5: Setting Realistic Recovery Goals

Recovering from an injury can be a long and challenging journey. Setting realistic goals can help you stay motivated and on track. Goals give you something to aim for and help measure your progress. This chapter will guide you on how to set realistic recovery goals that will help you heal effectively and get back to your normal activities.

Why Goals Are Important

Goals are like a roadmap for your recovery. They provide direction and keep you focused. When you set goals, you know what you are working towards and can see your progress along the way. This can be very motivating, especially when you're feeling down or frustrated. Goals also help you and your medical team create a clear plan for your recovery.

Understanding Your Injury
Before setting goals, it's important to understand your injury. Talk to your doctor or physical therapist to learn more about your injury and what to expect during your recovery. Ask questions like:

- How long will it take to heal?
- What activities should I avoid?
- What kind of exercises will help?

Having a clear understanding of your injury will help you set goals that are safe and achievable.

Setting Short-Term and Long-Term Goals
It's helpful to set both short-term and long-term goals. Short-term goals are things you can achieve in a few days or weeks. Long-term goals are bigger milestones that might take several months to reach.

Short-Term Goals

- Reduce pain and swelling
- Regain basic movement
- Start gentle exercises
- Follow your R.I.C.E. routine (Rest, Ice, Compression, Elevation)

Long-Term Goals

- Return to your favorite activities
- Regain full strength and flexibility
- Prevent future injuries

Making Your Goals SMART

A good way to set goals is to make them SMART: Specific, Measurable, Achievable, Relevant, and Time-bound.

Specific: Be clear about what you want to achieve. Instead of saying, "I want to get better," say, "I want to be able to walk without pain."

Measurable: Choose goals that you can measure. This helps you track your progress. For example, "I want to bend my knee 90 degrees" is a measurable goal.

Achievable: Set goals that are realistic. It's important to push yourself, but don't set goals that are too difficult or impossible. Talk to your doctor or therapist to make sure your goals are achievable.

Relevant: Your goals should be related to your recovery. Focus on what will help you heal and get back to your normal activities.

Time-bound: Set a timeline for your goals. This gives you a deadline and helps you stay focused. For example, "I want to walk without crutches in six weeks."

Creating an Action Plan

Once you have your goals, create an action plan. This is a step-by-step plan for how you will achieve your goals. Your action plan might include:

- Daily exercises and stretches
- Rest and recovery periods
- Regular check-ups with your doctor or therapist
- Healthy eating and hydration

Write down your action plan and keep it somewhere you can see it every day. This will remind you of what you need to do and keep you motivated.

Tracking Your Progress
Keep track of your progress by writing down your achievements. This can be in a notebook, a journal, or even a calendar. Note down when you reach a goal and how it makes you feel. Seeing your progress on paper can be very encouraging and help you stay positive.

Being Flexible

Recovery is not always a straight path. Sometimes, things don't go as planned, and that's okay. If you're not making the progress you hoped for, talk to your doctor or therapist. They can help you adjust your goals and action plan. Being flexible and willing to change your plan will help you stay on track.

Celebrating Your Successes

Celebrate your successes, no matter how small they may seem. Each step forward is a sign of progress. Treat yourself to something special when you reach a goal, whether it's a nice meal, a movie night, or something else you enjoy. Celebrating your achievements will boost your morale and keep you motivated.

Staying Positive and Patient

Recovering from an injury takes time, and it's important to stay positive and patient. There will be good days and bad days, but remember that every day is a step closer to your recovery. Surround yourself with supportive friends and family who can encourage you and help you stay motivated.

Setting realistic recovery goals is a crucial part of the healing process. Goals give you direction, keep you motivated, and help you measure your progress. By understanding your injury, setting SMART goals, creating an action plan, and tracking your progress, you can navigate your recovery journey with confidence. Stay positive, be patient, and celebrate each success along the way. With determination and the right goals, you'll be back to your normal activities and feeling stronger than ever.

Chapter 6: Importance of Rest and Recovery

When you're injured, rest and recovery are as important as any treatment or therapy. Taking the time to rest allows your body to heal and regain strength. This chapter will explain why rest is crucial, how it helps with recovery, and how to make the most of your rest periods. By understanding the importance of rest, you can help your body recover more effectively and get back to your regular activities sooner.

Why Rest is Crucial

When you get injured, your body needs time to repair itself. Resting gives your body the break it needs to focus on healing. During rest, your body can:

- Repair damaged tissues
- Reduce inflammation
- Rebuild strength and flexibility
- Prevent further injury

Without proper rest, you risk worsening your injury or causing new problems. Pushing yourself too hard can lead to setbacks and a longer recovery time.

How Rest Helps the Healing Process
Rest plays a vital role in each phase of the healing process. Let's take a closer look at how best supports each phase:

Inflammatory Phase: Right after an injury, your body goes into the inflammatory phase. During this time, rest helps reduce swelling and pain. It allows your body to send the necessary cells to the injured area to clean up damaged tissues and start the healing process.

Proliferative Phase: In this phase, your body starts building new tissues. Rest helps ensure that the new tissues form properly. Gentle movements recommended by your doctor or therapist can aid this process, but too much activity can disrupt the formation of new tissues.

Remodeling Phase: This final phase involves strengthening and fine-tuning the new tissues. Rest allows your body to focus on making these tissues as strong and functional as possible. Gradually increasing your activity levels under the guidance of a healthcare professional helps in this phase.

Different Types of Rest
Rest doesn't just mean lying in bed all day. There are different types of rest that can help you recover:

Active Rest: This involves gentle activities that don't strain the injured area. Walking, stretching, and light movements can help keep your body active without causing harm. Active rest promotes blood flow, which brings nutrients to the injured area and helps with healing.

Complete Rest: Sometimes, your body needs complete rest. This means avoiding any activity that might stress the injured area. Complete rest is crucial immediately after the injury and during times when the injury feels particularly painful or swollen.

Sleep: Sleep is one of the most important types of rest. During sleep, your body goes into repair mode. It produces growth hormones that help repair tissues and reduce inflammation. Aim for 7-9 hours of quality sleep each night to support your recovery.

Creating a Restful Environment

Creating a restful environment can help you make the most of your rest periods. Here are some tips to create a space that promotes healing:

- Comfortable Bed: Ensure your bed is comfortable and supportive. Use pillows to prop up the injured area and keep it elevated.
- Quiet Space: A quiet and peaceful environment helps you relax and get better sleep. Minimize noise and distractions, especially at night.
- Temperature: Keep your room at a comfortable temperature. Not too hot and not too cold.
- Relaxation Techniques: Practice relaxation techniques like deep breathing, meditation, or gentle stretching to reduce stress and promote healing.

Balancing Rest and Activity

While rest is crucial, it's also important to maintain some level of activity to prevent stiffness and muscle weakness. Balancing rest and activity can be tricky, but here are some guidelines:

- Follow Your Doctor's Advice: Your healthcare provider will give you specific instructions on how much rest and activity you need. Follow their advice carefully.
- Listen to Your Body: Pay attention to how your body feels. If you experience increased pain, swelling, or fatigue, it's a sign that you need more rest.
- Start Slow: When reintroducing activity, start with gentle movements and gradually increase your activity level. Don't rush the process.

Nutrition and Hydration

Rest and recovery are supported by good nutrition and hydration. Eating a balanced diet provides your body with the nutrients it needs to heal. Focus on foods rich in:

- Protein: Helps repair and build tissues. Good sources include lean meats, fish, beans, and nuts.
- Vitamins and Minerals: Support overall health and healing. Fruits, vegetables, and whole grains are excellent sources.
- Hydration: Drink plenty of water to stay hydrated. Water helps transport nutrients to the injured area and flushes out toxins.

Mental and Emotional Rest

Injury recovery is not just about physical rest; it's also about mental and emotional well-being. Stress and anxiety can slow down the healing process. Here are some ways to support your mental and emotional health during recovery:

- Stay Positive: Focus on your progress and celebrate small victories. Positive thinking can boost your mood and motivation.

- Connect with Others: Don't isolate yourself. Talk to friends and family, and share your feelings and experiences.
- Seek Support: Consider talking to a mental health professional if you're feeling overwhelmed. They can provide strategies to cope with stress and anxiety.

Rest and recovery are essential components of healing from an injury. By understanding the importance of rest and how it supports each phase of the healing process, you can make informed decisions about your recovery. Create a restful environment, balance rest and activity, and support your body with good nutrition and hydration. Remember to take care of your mental and emotional health as well. With proper rest and a positive mindset, you'll be on your way to a full and successful recovery.

Chapter 7: Nutrition for Healing

Eating the right foods is crucial when you're recovering from an injury. Good nutrition helps your body heal faster and get stronger. This chapter will explain how different nutrients support your recovery and provide tips on what to eat and drink. Understanding nutrition's role in healing will empower you to make better food choices that aid your recovery.

Why Nutrition Matters

When you're injured, your body needs extra nutrients to repair damaged tissues, reduce inflammation, and regain strength. Think of food as the fuel your body needs to get better. Eating the right foods can:

- Speed up the healing process
- Reduce inflammation
- Boost your immune system
- Restore energy levels
- Strengthen muscles and bones

Key Nutrients for Healing

Certain nutrients are especially important for healing. Let's look at some of these key nutrients and how they help your body recover.

Protein: Protein is the building block of your body. It helps repair tissues, build new cells, and strengthen muscles. Good sources of protein include:

- Lean meats like chicken, turkey, and beef
- Fish and seafood
- Eggs
- Dairy products like milk, yogurt, and cheese

- Plant-based proteins like beans, lentils, tofu, and nuts

Vitamin C: Vitamin C is essential for the production of collagen, a protein that helps rebuild skin, cartilage, and tendons. It also boosts your immune system and helps fight infections. Foods rich in vitamin C include:

- Citrus fruits like oranges, lemons, and grapefruits
- Berries like strawberries and blueberries
- Kiwi
- Bell peppers
- Broccoli and Brussels sprouts

Vitamin A: Vitamin A supports the growth and repair of tissues and helps maintain your immune system. You can find vitamin A in:

- Carrots
- Sweet potatoes

- Spinach and kale
- Red peppers
- Apricots

Zinc: Zinc plays a vital role in wound healing and immune function. Good sources of zinc are:

- Meat and poultry
- Seafood, especially oysters
- Dairy products
- Nuts and seeds
- Whole grains

Omega-3 Fatty Acids: Omega-3s help reduce inflammation and support tissue repair. You can get omega-3s from:

- Fatty fish like salmon, mackerel, and sardines
- Flaxseeds and chia seeds
- Walnuts
- Omega-3 fortified eggs

Calcium and Vitamin D: These nutrients are crucial for bone health and repair. Calcium-rich foods include:

- Dairy products like milk, cheese, and yogurt
- Leafy green vegetables like kale and broccoli
- Almonds
- Fortified plant-based milk (like almond or soy milk)

Vitamin D helps your body absorb calcium and can be found in:

- Fatty fish like salmon and tuna
- Egg yolks
- Fortified foods like milk and cereals
- Sunlight exposure (your body makes vitamin D when your skin is exposed to sunlight)

Hydration

Staying hydrated is just as important as eating the right foods. Water helps transport nutrients to your injured area, flush out toxins, and keep your tissues hydrated. Aim to drink at least 8 glasses of water a day, and more if you're active or it's hot outside. Other hydrating options include:

- Herbal teas
- Coconut water
- Broths and soups
- Water-rich fruits and vegetables like watermelon, cucumber, and oranges

Healthy Eating Tips

Here are some practical tips to help you eat well and support your recovery:

Eat a Balanced Diet: Include a variety of foods from all food groups: proteins, fruits, vegetables, grains, and dairy. This ensures you get a wide range of nutrients.

Don't Skip Meals: Regular meals provide a steady supply of nutrients. Try to eat three balanced meals a day and healthy snacks in between if needed.

Choose Whole Foods: Whole foods like fruits, vegetables, whole grains, and lean proteins are packed with nutrients. Avoid processed foods that are high in sugar, salt, and unhealthy fats.

Listen to Your Body: Pay attention to how different foods make you feel. If certain foods make you feel sluggish or uncomfortable, avoid them. Choose foods that give you energy and make you feel good.

Prepare Healthy Snacks: Keep healthy snacks on hand for when you're hungry between meals. Some good options include:

- Fresh fruit

- Yogurt with berries
- Nuts and seeds
- Whole grain crackers with cheese or hummus
- Veggie sticks with dip

Special Diet Considerations

If you have dietary restrictions or follow a special diet, you can still get the nutrients you need for healing. Here are some tips for different dietary needs:

Vegetarian/Vegan: Focus on plant-based proteins like beans, lentils, tofu, and tempeh. Include a variety of fruits, vegetables, nuts, seeds, and whole grains. Consider fortified foods or supplements for nutrients like vitamin B12, iron, and omega-3s.

Gluten-Free: Choose gluten-free grains like rice, quinoa, and corn. Many fruits, vegetables, proteins, and dairy products are naturally gluten-free. Be sure to read labels on packaged foods to avoid gluten.

Low-Lactose/Lactose-Free: Opt for lactose-free dairy products or plant-based alternatives like almond milk, soy yogurt, and coconut cheese. Include other calcium-rich foods like leafy greens, almonds, and fortified plant milks.

Meal Planning

Planning your meals ahead of time can help you make healthy choices and ensure you get all the nutrients you need. Here are some meal-planning tips:

- Plan for the Week: Take some time each week to plan your meals. Include a variety of proteins, fruits, vegetables, grains, and dairy.
- Prep Ahead: Prepare ingredients or cook meals in advance to save time during the week. For example, chop vegetables, cook grains, or make a big batch of soup.

- Healthy Recipes: Look for healthy recipes that are easy to make and include healing nutrients. There are many resources online with delicious and nutritious meal ideas.
- Portion Control: Be mindful of portion sizes to avoid overeating. Use smaller plates and listen to your body's hunger and fullness cues.

Supplements

Sometimes, it can be hard to get all the nutrients you need from food alone, especially if you have dietary restrictions. Supplements can help fill the gaps. Talk to your doctor before taking any supplements to make sure they're safe and appropriate for you. Some common supplements for healing include:

- Multivitamins: A good multivitamin can provide a variety of essential nutrients.

- Protein Powder: Protein powder can be an easy way to boost your protein intake, especially if you're not getting enough from food.
- Vitamin C and Zinc: These supplements can support your immune system and help with tissue repair.
- Omega-3s: Fish oil or flaxseed oil supplements can provide omega-3 fatty acids.

Nutrition plays a crucial role in your recovery from injury. By eating a balanced diet rich in key nutrients, staying hydrated, and making healthy food choices, you can support your body's healing process. Pay attention to your body's needs, plan your meals, and consider supplements if necessary. With the right nutrition, you'll be on your way to a faster and stronger recovery.

Chapter 8: Pain Management Techniques

Dealing with pain is a common part of recovering from an injury. Managing pain effectively can make a big difference in your recovery process. This chapter will explore various pain management techniques, from medication to natural methods, to help you find relief and heal more comfortably. Understanding these techniques will empower you to handle pain better and speed up your recovery.

Understanding Pain

Pain is your body's way of signaling that something is wrong. It's an important protective mechanism, but it can also be very uncomfortable and frustrating. There are two main types of pain you might experience:

- Acute Pain: This is short-term pain that comes on suddenly and usually has a clear cause, like an injury. It tends to improve as your injury heals.
- Chronic Pain: This is long-term pain that persists for months or even years. It can be caused by ongoing issues like arthritis or nerve damage.

Knowing what type of pain you're dealing with can help you choose the best pain management techniques.

Medication for Pain Relief

One of the most common ways to manage pain is through medication. There are several types of pain relief medications, each working in different ways. Always follow your doctor's advice when taking medication.

Over-the-Counter Pain Relievers

- Acetaminophen (Tylenol): This medication can help reduce pain and fever. It's generally safe when taken as directed.
- Nonsteroidal Anti-Inflammatory Drugs (NSAIDs): These include ibuprofen (Advil, Motrin) and naproxen (Aleve). They help reduce pain, inflammation, and swelling. Be cautious with long-term use, as they can cause stomach problems.

Prescription Medications
- Stronger NSAIDs: Sometimes, doctors prescribe stronger NSAIDs for more severe pain.
- Opioids: These are powerful pain relievers used for severe pain. They can be very effective but come with risks of addiction and side effects. They should be used only as prescribed and under close supervision.
- Muscle Relaxants: These can help if your pain is related to muscle spasms.
- Topical Pain Relievers: These creams or gels are applied directly to the skin over the painful area.

They can provide targeted relief without many of the side effects of oral medications.

Natural Pain Relief Methods

There are many natural ways to manage pain that can be used alone or along with medication. These methods often have fewer side effects and can be very effective.

Rest and Ice

- Rest: Giving your body time to heal is crucial. Avoid activities that cause pain and allow your injury to recover.
- Ice: Applying ice to the injured area can reduce pain and swelling. Use an ice pack wrapped in a cloth for 15-20 minutes every few hours.

Heat Therapy

- Heat: Applying heat can relax muscles and improve blood flow. Use a warm towel or heating pad on the painful area for 15-20 minutes. Be careful not to burn your skin.

Physical Therapy
- Exercises: Physical therapists can teach you exercises that strengthen the injured area and improve flexibility, reducing pain.
- Manual Therapy: Techniques like massage or joint manipulation can help relieve pain and improve movement.

Relaxation Techniques
- Deep Breathing: Taking slow, deep breaths can help you relax and reduce pain.
- Meditation: Practicing mindfulness or meditation can help you manage pain by focusing your mind away from the discomfort.

Acupuncture
- Acupuncture: This traditional Chinese medicine technique involves inserting thin needles into

specific points on your body. It can help reduce pain and promote healing.

Chiropractic Care
- Chiropractic Adjustments: Chiropractors can adjust your spine and joints to improve alignment and reduce pain.

TENS Therapy
- Transcutaneous Electrical Nerve Stimulation (TENS): This involves using a small device that sends electrical impulses to the painful area, which can help reduce pain signals.

Lifestyle Changes for Pain Management
Making certain lifestyle changes can also help you manage pain more effectively.
Healthy Diet
- Nutrition: Eating a balanced diet rich in anti-inflammatory foods like fruits, vegetables, whole

grains, and lean proteins can help reduce pain and promote healing.

Regular Exercise
- Exercise: Staying active, and within your limits, can help keep your body strong and reduce pain. Low-impact activities like walking, swimming, and yoga are good options.

Adequate Sleep
- Sleep: Getting enough sleep is essential for healing and pain management. Aim for 7-9 hours of quality sleep each night. Create a relaxing bedtime routine and make your sleep environment comfortable.

Stress Management
- Stress Reduction: Stress can make pain worse. Find ways to relax and reduce stress, such as spending time with loved ones, hobbies, or listening to music.

Support and Communication

Having a support system and communicating with your healthcare team are vital parts of managing pain.

Support System

- Friends and Family: Let your friends and family know how they can support you. Sometimes just talking about your pain can help you feel better.
- Support Groups: Joining a support group for people with similar injuries or pain can provide emotional support and practical advice.

Communication with Healthcare Providers

- Talk to Your Doctor: Keep your doctor informed about your pain levels and how different treatments are working. They can adjust your treatment plan as needed.

- Follow-Up Appointments: Attend all follow-up appointments to track your progress and make necessary changes to your pain management plan.

Managing pain effectively is crucial for a smooth and successful recovery. Whether through medication, natural methods, lifestyle changes, or a combination of these, there are many ways to find relief. By understanding the different pain management techniques and working closely with your healthcare team, you can handle pain better and focus on healing. Remember, everyone's pain experience is different, so find the methods that work best for you and stick with them. With the right approach, you can manage your pain and get back to enjoying life.

Chapter 9: The Benefits of Physical Therapy

Recovering from an injury can be challenging, but physical therapy (PT) can make the journey smoother and faster. Physical therapy involves exercises and treatments designed to help you regain movement, strength, and function. This chapter will explore the many benefits of physical therapy and how it can aid your recovery. By understanding the role of PT, you can take advantage of this valuable resource and improve your healing process.

What is Physical Therapy?
Physical therapy is a type of healthcare that helps you recover from injuries, manage pain, and improve your physical abilities. Physical therapists are trained professionals who create personalized

treatment plans based on your specific needs and goals. PT can include a variety of techniques such as exercises, stretches, manual therapy, and the use of equipment to help you get better.

Benefits of Physical Therapy

Physical therapy offers numerous benefits that can enhance your recovery and overall well-being. Let's dive into some of the key benefits.

1. Pain Relief

One of the primary benefits of physical therapy is pain relief. Physical therapists use different techniques to reduce pain, including:

- Manual Therapy: Hands-on techniques like massage and joint mobilization to ease pain and improve movement.
- Modalities: Treatments such as heat, ice, ultrasound, and electrical stimulation to reduce pain and inflammation.

2. Improved Mobility and Flexibility

Injuries can make it hard to move and do everyday activities. Physical therapy helps you regain mobility and flexibility through:

- Stretching Exercises: Specific stretches to improve the range of motion in your joints and muscles.
- Strengthening Exercises: Exercises to build strength in the muscles around your injury, providing better support and stability.

3. Faster Recovery

Physical therapy can speed up your recovery by promoting healing and preventing complications. With a personalized PT plan, you can:

- Target Weak Areas: Strengthen and stabilize the injured area, making it less prone to re-injury.

- Improve Circulation: Exercises that increase blood flow to the injured area, delivering more oxygen and nutrients needed for healing.

4. Prevention of Future Injuries

A significant advantage of physical therapy is learning how to avoid future injuries. Physical therapists teach you:

- Proper Techniques: How to move and exercise safely to prevent re-injury.
- Body Mechanics: Ways to use your body correctly during activities and sports to reduce strain and risk of injury.

5. Better Balance and Coordination

After an injury, your balance and coordination can be affected. Physical therapy helps you regain these essential skills through:

- Balance Exercises: Activities that challenge your balance and help you regain stability.
- Coordination Training: Exercises that improve the coordination between your muscles and nerves, helping you move more efficiently.

6. Personalized Care

One of the best things about physical therapy is that it's tailored to your needs. Your physical therapist will:

- Assess Your Condition: Evaluate your injury and create a treatment plan specific to your situation.
- Monitor Progress: Adjust your exercises and treatments as you improve to ensure you're always moving forward.

7. Non-Invasive Treatment

Physical therapy is a non-invasive treatment option that can often help you avoid surgery or reduce the need for medication. By using natural healing methods like exercise and manual therapy, PT promotes recovery without the risks associated with surgery or long-term medication use.

8. Education and Empowerment

Physical therapy empowers you by teaching you about your body and how to care for it. You'll learn:

- Injury Prevention: How to prevent future injuries through proper techniques and exercises.
- Self-Management: Strategies to manage pain and maintain your progress even after your PT sessions are over.

Types of Physical Therapy

There are different types of physical therapy tailored to various needs and conditions. Here are a few common types:

Orthopedic Physical Therapy: Focuses on musculoskeletal injuries like fractures, sprains, and arthritis. It helps improve mobility, strength, and function in bones, muscles, and joints.

Neurological Physical Therapy: Aims to improve movement and function in individuals with neurological conditions like stroke, Parkinson's disease, or spinal cord injuries.

Cardiopulmonary Physical Therapy: Helps individuals with heart and lung conditions improve their cardiovascular health and endurance.

Pediatric Physical Therapy: Designed for children with injuries or developmental issues to enhance their physical abilities and overall growth.

Geriatric Physical Therapy: Focuses on the needs of older adults, addressing age-related conditions like osteoporosis and arthritis to improve mobility and quality of life.

What to Expect in Physical Therapy
Starting physical therapy can feel overwhelming, but knowing what to expect can make it easier. Here's a typical PT journey:

Initial Assessment: Your physical therapist will conduct a thorough evaluation, asking about your medical history, symptoms, and goals. They may also perform physical tests to assess your strength, mobility, and pain levels.

Personalized Treatment Plan: Based on the assessment, your therapist will create a treatment plan tailored to your needs. This plan will include specific exercises and techniques to help you recover.

Regular Sessions: You'll attend regular PT sessions, where your therapist will guide you through exercises and treatments. They'll monitor your progress and adjust the plan as needed.

Home Exercises: Your therapist will likely give you exercises to do at home to complement your in-session work. Consistency is key to making steady progress.

Ongoing Support: Throughout your PT journey, your therapist will provide support, answer your questions, and ensure you're on the right track to recovery.

Physical therapy offers numerous benefits that can significantly improve your recovery and quality of life. From pain relief and improved mobility to faster recovery and injury prevention, PT provides a comprehensive approach to healing. By working with a skilled physical therapist and following a personalized treatment plan, you can overcome your injury and get back to doing the things you love. Embrace the journey and take advantage of the many benefits physical therapy has to offer.

Chapter 10: Developing a Rehabilitation Plan

Creating a rehabilitation plan is a crucial step in recovering from an injury. A well-thought-out plan helps you regain strength, mobility, and function, guiding you back to your normal activities. This chapter will explain how to develop an effective rehab plan, the key components involved, and how to stick with it for the best results. Understanding and following a rehabilitation plan can make your recovery smoother and more successful.

The Importance of a Rehabilitation Plan
When you're injured, your body needs time and proper care to heal. A rehabilitation plan provides a structured approach to recovery, ensuring you're doing the right exercises and activities to support healing. Without a plan, it's easy to either overdo it

and risk further injury or underdo it and delay your progress. A good rehab plan helps you find the right balance.

Steps to Develop a Rehabilitation Plan
Developing a rehab plan involves several important steps. Let's go through each step to understand how to create a plan that works for you.

1. Get a Professional Assessment
The first step in developing a rehabilitation plan is to get a professional assessment. Visit a healthcare provider, such as a doctor or physical therapist, who can evaluate your injury. They will:

- Examine your injury and assess its severity
- Discuss your medical history and any previous injuries
- Understand your goals and daily activities

This assessment provides a clear picture of your condition and helps in creating a personalized rehab plan.

2. Set Clear Goals

Setting clear, realistic goals is essential for a successful rehabilitation plan. Goals give you something to work towards and help you track your progress. Your goals should be:

- Specific: Clearly define what you want to achieve, such as regaining full range of motion in your knee or being able to walk without pain.
- Measurable: Ensure your goals are measurable so you can track your progress. For example, being able to walk a certain distance or lift a specific weight.
- Achievable: Set goals that are challenging but realistic, considering your current condition.
- Relevant: Make sure your goals are relevant to your daily activities and overall recovery.

- Time-bound: Set a timeline for achieving your goals, such as being able to jog again within three months.

3. Create a Personalized Exercise Program

Exercises are a core part of any rehabilitation plan. Your healthcare provider or physical therapist will design a personalized exercise program tailored to your needs. This program will likely include:

- Stretching Exercises: To improve flexibility and range of motion in the injured area.
- Strengthening Exercises: To build strength in the muscles around the injury, providing better support and stability.
- Cardiovascular Exercises: To maintain overall fitness and support circulation, which helps with healing.
- Balance and Coordination Exercises: To regain stability and coordination, especially if your injury affects your balance.

4. Incorporate Rest and Recovery

Rest and recovery are just as important as exercise in a rehab plan. Your body needs time to heal and repair itself. Incorporate rest days into your plan to avoid overtraining and further injury. Listen to your body and give it the rest it needs.

5. Monitor Your Progress

Keeping track of your progress helps you stay motivated and see how far you've come. Regularly assess your improvement and adjust your plan as needed. You can:

- Keep a journal or log of your exercises and progress
- Take notes on pain levels, range of motion, and strength gains
- Share your progress with your healthcare provider or physical therapist during follow-up visits

6. Stay Consistent and Motivated

Sticking to your rehab plan is crucial for recovery. Consistency is key, but it's also important to stay motivated. Here are some tips to help you stay on track:

- Set Small Milestones: Break your larger goals into smaller, achievable milestones. Celebrate these small victories to stay motivated.
- Find a Support System: Share your goals with friends, family, or a support group. Having others cheer you on can boost your motivation.
- Mix It Up: Variety in your exercises can keep things interesting. Try different activities to avoid getting bored.
- Stay Positive: Focus on the progress you've made rather than the setbacks. A positive mindset can make a big difference.

7. Adjust Your Plan as Needed

Recovery is not always a straight path. You might face setbacks or challenges along the way. It's important to be flexible and adjust your plan as needed. Work with your healthcare provider or physical therapist to make any necessary changes based on your progress and how your body is responding.

Developing a rehabilitation plan is a crucial step in recovering from an injury. By getting a professional assessment, setting clear goals, creating a personalized exercise program, incorporating rest, monitoring progress, staying consistent and motivated, and adjusting the plan as needed, you can enhance your recovery and regain your strength and mobility. Remember, a good rehab plan is tailored to your needs and helps you achieve your goals step by step. With dedication and the right plan, you can overcome your injury and get back to your normal activities.

Chapter 11: Stretching and Flexibility Exercises

Stretching and flexibility exercises are vital parts of any rehabilitation plan. They help improve your range of motion, reduce stiffness, and prevent future injuries. This chapter will explain the importance of stretching, the different types of stretches, and how to incorporate them into your daily routine. By the end, you'll understand how to use these exercises to aid your recovery and enhance your overall physical health.

Why Stretching and Flexibility Are Important
When you're injured, the affected area often becomes stiff and tight. Stretching helps to:

- Improve Range of Motion: Stretching allows your joints and muscles to move more freely, making everyday activities easier.
- Reduce Pain and Stiffness: Regular stretching can alleviate pain and discomfort associated with tight muscles.
- Prevent Future Injuries: Keeping your muscles flexible reduces the risk of strains and sprains.
- Enhance Blood Flow: Stretching improves circulation, delivering more oxygen and nutrients to your muscles, which aids in healing.
- Improve Posture: Stretching can correct imbalances and improve your posture, reducing the strain on your body.

Types of Stretching Exercises

There are several types of stretching exercises, each serving a different purpose. Understanding these can help you choose the best ones for your rehabilitation.

1. Static Stretching

Static stretching involves holding a stretch for a period, usually between 15-60 seconds. This type of stretching is great for improving flexibility and should be done after your muscles are warmed up. Examples include:

- Hamstring Stretch: Sit on the floor with one leg extended and the other bent. Reach toward your toes on the extended leg and hold.
- Quadriceps Stretch: Stand on one leg, grab your opposite ankle, and pull it towards your buttocks, holding the stretch.

2. Dynamic Stretching

Dynamic stretching involves moving parts of your body through a full range of motion. This type of stretching is good for warming up before physical activity. Examples include:

- Leg Swings: Stand on one leg and swing the other leg forward and backward, gradually increasing the range of motion.
- Arm Circles: Extend your arms to the sides and make small circles, gradually increasing their size.

3. PNF Stretching

Proprioceptive Neuromuscular Facilitation (PNF) stretching involves alternating between stretching and contracting the muscle. It's often done with a partner. Examples include:

- Hamstring PNF Stretch: Lie on your back and raise one leg. Have a partner push it toward your chest while you resist slightly. Relax and then stretch further.

4. Active Stretching

Active stretching involves using your muscles to hold a stretch position without any assistance. This helps build strength and flexibility. Examples include:

- Standing Calf Stretch: Stand with one foot forward and one foot back, pressing your heel into the ground to stretch your calf.
- Seated Forward Bend: Sit with your legs extended and reach forward to touch your toes, engaging your core muscles.

How to Incorporate Stretching into Your Routine
Incorporating stretching into your daily routine can significantly enhance your recovery. Here's how to do it effectively:

1. Warm Up First
Always warm up your muscles before stretching. A light activity like walking or gentle cycling for 5-10 minutes can increase blood flow and make your muscles more pliable.

2. Stretch Regularly

Consistency is key. Aim to stretch every day, especially the muscles around your injured area. You don't need to spend hours; even 10-15 minutes a day can make a big difference.

3. Listen to Your Body

Stretching should feel good, not painful. You might feel a gentle pull, but if you experience sharp pain, stop immediately. Stretch within your comfort zone and gradually increase the intensity as your flexibility improves.

4. Breathe Deeply

Breathing deeply and slowly helps relax your muscles and improve the effectiveness of your stretches. Focus on your breath as you hold each stretch.

5. Use Proper Technique

Proper technique is crucial to avoid further injury. Here are some tips:

- Move smoothly and avoid bouncing.
- Hold each stretch for the recommended time.
- Keep your movements controlled and deliberate.

Sample Stretching Routine

Here's a simple stretching routine you can follow to improve your flexibility and support your rehabilitation:

1. Neck Stretch: Sit or stand up straight. Slowly tilt your head to one side, bringing your ear toward your shoulder. Hold for 15-30 seconds, then switch sides.
2. Shoulder Stretch: Bring one arm across your chest and use your opposite hand to gently pull it closer. Hold for 15-30 seconds, then switch arms.
3. Triceps Stretch: Raise one arm overhead and bend your elbow, reaching down your back. Use

your other hand to gently push your elbow. Hold for 15-30 seconds, then switch arms.

4. Chest Stretch: Stand in a doorway with your arms at a 90-degree angle, hands against the doorframe. Step forward until you feel a stretch in your chest. Hold for 15-30 seconds.

5. Hamstring Stretch: Sit on the floor with one leg extended and the other bent. Reach toward your toes on the extended leg and hold for 15-30 seconds, then switch legs.

6. Quad Stretch: Stand on one leg, grab your opposite ankle, and pull it towards your buttocks. Hold for 15-30 seconds, then switch legs.

7. Calf Stretch: Stand facing a wall with one foot forward and the other back. Press your back heel into the ground, feeling the stretch in your calf. Hold for 15-30 seconds, then switch legs.

Staying Motivated

Sticking to a stretching routine can sometimes be challenging. Here are some tips to stay motivated:

- Set Goals: Set small, achievable goals for your flexibility and celebrate your progress.
- Make It Enjoyable: Listen to music or a podcast while you stretch to make it more enjoyable.
- Track Your Progress: Keep a journal or take photos to see how your flexibility improves over time.
- Get Support: Join a stretching class or find a stretching partner to keep you accountable.

Stretching and flexibility exercises are essential components of a successful rehabilitation plan. They help improve your range of motion, reduce pain and stiffness, and prevent future injuries. By incorporating regular stretching into your routine and following the right techniques, you can enhance your recovery and overall physical health. Remember, consistency is key, so make stretching a daily habit. With dedication and patience, you'll see significant improvements in your flexibility and overall well-being.

Chapter 12: Strength Training for Recovery

Strength training is an essential part of recovering from an injury. It helps rebuild muscle, improve stability, and prevent future injuries. This chapter will explain the importance of strength training, how to safely incorporate it into your rehabilitation plan, and the different types of exercises you can do. By the end, you'll understand how to use strength training to speed up your recovery and enhance your overall health.

Why Strength Training is Important

When you're injured, the muscles around the affected area can weaken. Strength training helps:

- Rebuild Muscle: Injuries often cause muscle loss. Strength training rebuilds these muscles, helping you regain your strength.
- Improve Stability: Strong muscles support your joints and improve your balance, reducing the risk of future injuries.
- Enhance Mobility: Strengthening exercises can improve your range of motion and make daily activities easier.
- Speed-Up Recovery: Building muscle can promote faster healing by increasing blood flow and nutrients to the injured area.
- Boost Confidence: As you get stronger, you'll feel more confident in your abilities and less afraid of re-injury.

Steps to Start Strength Training

Starting strength training can seem daunting, especially after an injury. Follow these steps to ensure you do it safely and effectively.

1. Get a Professional Assessment

Before starting any strength training, consult with a healthcare provider or physical therapist. They can:

- Evaluate your injury and overall fitness level
- Identify which muscles need strengthening
- Create a personalized strength training plan

2. Set Clear Goals

Having clear goals helps you stay focused and motivated. Your goals should be:

- Specific: Clearly define what you want to achieve, such as being able to lift a certain weight or perform a specific exercise.
- Measurable: Make sure your goals can be tracked, like increasing the number of repetitions or sets.
- Achievable: Set realistic goals based on your current condition.
- Relevant: Ensure your goals are related to your recovery needs.

- Time-bound: Set a timeline for achieving your goals.

3. Start with Low-Impact Exercises

Begin with low-impact exercises that are gentle on your injury. These exercises build a foundation of strength without putting too much strain on your body. Examples include:

- Bodyweight Exercises: Squats, lunges, and push-ups use your body weight to build strength.
- Resistance Bands: These provide gentle resistance, making them ideal for beginners.
- Water Exercises: Swimming and water aerobics reduce stress on your joints while building strength.

4. Gradually Increase Intensity

As your strength improves, gradually increase the intensity of your workouts. This can be done by:

- Increasing the weight or resistance

- Adding more repetitions or sets
- Trying more challenging exercises

Always listen to your body and avoid pushing too hard too soon. Gradual progression is key to preventing further injury.

5. Focus on Proper Form

Proper form is crucial to avoid injury and get the most out of your exercises. Here are some tips:

- Move Slowly: Perform each exercise slowly and with control.
- Use the Right Muscles: Focus on engaging the correct muscles for each exercise.
- Avoid Cheating: Don't use momentum or other muscles to compensate for weakness.

If you're unsure about your form, ask a physical therapist or trainer for guidance.

6. Include Rest Days

Rest is just as important as exercise in strength training. Your muscles need time to recover and grow stronger. Include rest days in your training plan to prevent overtraining and further injury.

Types of Strength Training Exercises
There are various types of strength training exercises, each targeting different muscle groups. Here are some common exercises to include in your routine:

Upper Body Exercises
- Push-Ups: Great for building strength in your chest, shoulders, and triceps.
- Dumbbell Rows: Strengthen your back and biceps by lifting a dumbbell towards your chest while bent over.
- Shoulder Press: Press dumbbells or a barbell overhead to build shoulder strength.

Lower Body Exercises

- Squats: Strengthen your thighs, hips, and buttocks by bending your knees and lowering your body.
- Lunges: Step forward and lower your body to build strength in your legs and hips.
- Leg Press: Use a leg press machine to target your quadriceps, hamstrings, and glutes.

Core Exercises
- Planks: Hold a plank position to strengthen your core muscles.
- Russian Twists: Sit on the floor, lean back slightly, and twist your torso to work your obliques.
- Bicycle Crunches: Lie on your back, lift your legs, and alternate bringing your knees to your elbows to target your abs.

Creating a Balanced Strength Training Routine

A balanced routine includes exercises for all major muscle groups and incorporates different types of strength training. Here's an example of a weekly routine:

Day 1: Upper Body
- Push-Ups: 3 sets of 10-15 reps
- Dumbbell Rows: 3 sets of 10-15 reps
- Shoulder Press: 3 sets of 10-15 reps

Day 2: Lower Body
- Squats: 3 sets of 10-15 reps
- Lunges: 3 sets of 10-15 reps (each leg)
- Leg Press: 3 sets of 10-15 reps

Day 3: Core
- Planks: 3 sets of 30-60 seconds
- Russian Twists: 3 sets of 15-20 reps
- Bicycle Crunches: 3 sets of 15-20 reps

Day 4: Rest

Day 5: Full Body

- Push-Ups: 3 sets of 10-15 reps
- Squats: 3 sets of 10-15 reps
- Planks: 3 sets of 30-60 seconds

Day 6: Active Recovery
- Gentle yoga or stretching
- Light walking or swimming

Day 7: Rest

Staying Motivated

Staying motivated can be challenging, especially during recovery. Here are some tips to keep you on track:

- Track Your Progress: Keep a journal or use an app to track your workouts and progress.
- Set Short-Term Goals: Break your long-term goals into smaller, achievable milestones.

- Find a Workout Buddy: Exercising with a friend can make workouts more enjoyable and keep you accountable.
- Celebrate Achievements: Reward yourself when you reach your goals, no matter how small.

Strength training is a vital component of injury recovery. It helps rebuild muscle, improve stability, enhance mobility, and prevent future injuries. By getting a professional assessment, setting clear goals, starting with low-impact exercises, gradually increasing intensity, focusing on proper form, including rest days, and staying motivated, you can effectively use strength training to speed up your recovery. Remember, consistency and patience are key. With the right approach, you can regain your strength and get back to doing the things you love.

Chapter 13: Cardiovascular Conditioning

Cardiovascular conditioning is a key part of recovery from an injury. It helps improve your heart and lung function, increases your stamina, and aids in overall fitness. This chapter will explain why cardiovascular conditioning is important, how to safely incorporate it into your rehabilitation plan, and the different types of cardio exercises you can do. By the end, you'll understand how to use cardiovascular conditioning to support your recovery and enhance your health.

Why Cardiovascular Conditioning is Important

When you're injured, it's easy to become less active, which can lead to a decline in cardiovascular fitness. Cardiovascular conditioning helps:

- Improve Heart and Lung Health: Regular cardio exercises strengthen your heart and lungs, making them more efficient.
- Increase Stamina: Cardio workouts boost your endurance, allowing you to perform daily activities with less fatigue.
- Aid in Weight Management: Cardio exercises burn calories, helping you maintain a healthy weight, which reduces stress on your joints.
- Enhance Mood: Physical activity releases endorphins, which can improve your mood and reduce stress.
- Promote Faster Healing: Improved blood circulation from cardio exercises helps deliver oxygen and nutrients to injured tissues, speeding up the healing process.

Steps to Start Cardiovascular Conditioning

Starting cardiovascular conditioning can be challenging, especially after an injury. Follow these steps to ensure you do it safely and effectively.

1. Consult a Healthcare Provider

Before beginning any cardio exercises, consult with a healthcare provider or physical therapist. They can:

- Assess your injury and overall fitness level
- Identify safe cardio exercises for your condition
- Create a personalized cardio plan

2. Set Realistic Goals

Setting realistic goals helps you stay focused and motivated. Your goals should be:

- Specific: Clearly define what you want to achieve, such as walking a certain distance or duration.

- Measurable: Make sure your goals can be tracked, like increasing your walking time by a few minutes each week.
- Achievable: Set realistic goals based on your current fitness level and injury status.
- Relevant: Ensure your goals are related to your recovery and overall fitness.
- Time-bound: Set a timeline for achieving your goals.

3. Start with Low-Impact Exercises

Begin with low-impact cardio exercises that are gentle on your injury. These exercises provide a cardiovascular workout without putting too much strain on your body. Examples include:

- Walking: Walking is a simple, effective way to start cardio conditioning. Begin with short walks and gradually increase your distance and pace.

- Swimming: Swimming is excellent for cardio because it supports your body and reduces stress on your joints.
- Cycling: Stationary cycling or riding a bike can provide a good cardio workout without excessive impact on your joints.

4. Gradually Increase Intensity

As your cardiovascular fitness improves, gradually increase the intensity of your workouts. This can be done by:

- Increasing the duration of your exercise sessions
- Adding intervals of higher intensity (e.g., brisk walking mixed with regular walking)
- Trying more challenging exercises

Always listen to your body and avoid pushing too hard too soon. Gradual progression is key to preventing further injury.

5. Monitor Your Heart Rate

Monitoring your heart rate during cardio exercises helps ensure you're working at the right intensity. Here's how to do it:

- Find Your Target Heart Rate: Your target heart rate is 50-70% of your maximum heart rate (220 minus your age).
- Use a Heart Rate Monitor: A heart rate monitor can help you stay within your target range.
- Check Your Pulse: You can also check your pulse manually by placing your fingers on your wrist or neck.

Types of Cardiovascular Exercises

There are various types of cardio exercises you can include in your routine. Here are some common options:

Low-Impact Exercises

- Walking: Start with 10-15 minutes and gradually increase your time.
- Swimming: Swim laps or do water aerobics for 20-30 minutes.
- Cycling: Use a stationary bike or ride a bike outside for 20-30 minutes.

Moderate-Impact Exercises
- Elliptical Trainer: Use an elliptical machine for a low-impact, full-body workout.
- Rowing Machine: Rowing provides a good cardio workout while being easy on the joints.
- Dance: Join a dance class or follow a dance workout video for a fun cardio session.

High-Impact Exercises (once you're ready)
- Running: Start with short, easy runs and gradually increase your distance and speed.
- Jump Rope: Jumping rope is a high-impact cardio exercise that can be done in short bursts.

- High-Intensity Interval Training (HIIT):** Alternate between short periods of intense activity and rest.

Creating a Balanced Cardio Routine

A balanced cardio routine includes different types of exercises and varying intensities. Here's an example of a weekly routine:

Day 1: Walking
- Walk for 20-30 minutes at a comfortable pace.

Day 2: Swimming
- Swim laps or do water aerobics for 20-30 minutes.

Day 3: Rest

Day 4: Cycling
- Cycle on a stationary bike or ride outside for 20-30 minutes.

Day 5: Elliptical Trainer
- Use an elliptical machine for 20-30 minutes.

Day 6: Dance
- Follow a dance workout video or join a class for 20-30 minutes.

Day 7: Rest

Staying Motivated

Staying motivated can be challenging, especially during recovery. Here are some tips to keep you on track:

- Track Your Progress: Keep a journal or use an app to log your workouts and progress.
- Set Short-Term Goals: Break your long-term goals into smaller, achievable milestones.
- Find a Workout Buddy: Exercising with a friend can make workouts more enjoyable and keep you accountable.

- Celebrate Achievements: Reward yourself when you reach your goals, no matter how small.

Cardiovascular conditioning is a crucial part of injury recovery. It helps improve heart and lung function, increase stamina, manage weight, enhance mood, and promote faster healing. By consulting a healthcare provider, setting realistic goals, starting with low-impact exercises, gradually increasing intensity, monitoring your heart rate, and staying motivated, you can effectively use cardio exercises to support your recovery. Remember, consistency and patience are key. With the right approach, you can regain your cardiovascular fitness and get back to enjoying your favorite activities.

Chapter 14: Balance and Coordination Exercises

Balance and coordination exercises are essential for recovering from an injury. They help improve your stability, prevent future injuries, and make daily activities easier. This chapter will explain why balance and coordination are important, how to safely incorporate these exercises into your rehabilitation plan, and different exercises you can try. By the end, you'll understand how to use balance and coordination exercises to support your recovery and enhance your overall health.

Why Balance and Coordination Are Important
When you're injured, your body's balance and coordination can be affected. Working on these areas helps:

- Improve Stability: Good balance helps you stay steady on your feet, reducing the risk of falls and further injuries.

- Enhance Coordination: Improved coordination makes everyday activities like walking, reaching, and bending easier and safer.

- Strengthen Muscles: Balance exercises engage and strengthen the muscles around your joints.

- Boost Confidence: As your balance and coordination improve, you'll feel more confident in your movements and less fearful of re-injury.

- Prevent Future Injuries: A well-balanced body is less likely to suffer from strains and sprains.

Steps to Start Balance and Coordination Exercises

Starting balance and coordination exercises can be challenging, especially after an injury. Follow these steps to ensure you do it safely and effectively.

1. Consult a Healthcare Provider

Before beginning any balance and coordination exercises, consult with a healthcare provider or physical therapist. They can:

- Assess your injury and overall fitness level
- Identify safe exercises for your condition
- Create a personalized exercise plan

2. Set Clear Goals

Setting clear goals helps you stay focused and motivated. Your goals should be:

- Specific: Clearly define what you want to achieve, such as standing on one leg for a certain amount of time.
- Measurable: Make sure your goals can be tracked, like increasing the duration or difficulty of your exercises.
- Achievable: Set realistic goals based on your current condition.

- Relevant: Ensure your goals are related to your recovery and overall balance and coordination.
- Time-bound: Set a timeline for achieving your goals.

3. Start with Simple Exercises

Begin with simple balance and coordination exercises that are gentle on your injury. These exercises build a foundation of stability without putting too much strain on your body. Examples include:

- Standing on One Leg: Stand on one leg for 10-30 seconds, then switch legs. Use a chair or wall for support if needed.
- Heel-to-Toe Walk: Walk in a straight line, placing the heel of one foot directly in front of the toes of the other foot.
- Seated March: Sit on a chair and lift one knee at a time, as if marching in place.

4. Gradually Increase Difficulty

As your balance and coordination improve, gradually increase the difficulty of your exercises. This can be done by:

- Extending the duration of each exercise
- Performing exercises on an unstable surface (like a balance pad or pillow)
- Incorporating movement (like reaching or turning) into your exercises

Always listen to your body and avoid pushing too hard too soon. Gradual progression is key to preventing further injury.

5. Focus on Proper Form

Proper form is crucial to avoid injury and get the most out of your exercises. Here are some tips:

- Engage Your Core: Keep your abdominal muscles tight to help stabilize your body.

- Stay Upright: Maintain good posture by keeping your back straight and shoulders relaxed.
- Move Slowly: Perform each exercise slowly and with control to maximize the benefits.

Types of Balance and Coordination Exercises

There are various types of balance and coordination exercises you can include in your routine. Here are some common options:

Basic Balance Exercises

- Standing on One Leg: Stand on one leg for 10-30 seconds, then switch legs.
- Heel-to-Toe Walk: Walk in a straight line, placing the heel of one foot directly in front of the toes of the other foot.
- Seated March: Sit on a chair and lift one knee at a time, as if marching in place.

Intermediate Balance Exercises

- Balance on an Unstable Surface: Stand on a balance pad, pillow, or foam roller to challenge your stability.
- Single-Leg Deadlift: Stand on one leg and bend forward at the hips, reaching towards the ground, then return to standing.
- Side Leg Lift: Stand on one leg and lift the other leg to the side, then return to the starting position. Switch legs and repeat.

Advanced Balance Exercises
- Bosu Ball Squats: Stand on a Bosu ball and perform squats, maintaining your balance.
- Tandem Stand with Eyes Closed: Stand with one foot in front of the other, close your eyes, and hold your balance.
- Tai Chi: Practice Tai Chi movements, which emphasize slow, controlled motions and balance.

Creating a Balanced Routine

A balanced routine includes different types of exercises and varying difficulties. Here's an example of a weekly routine:

Day 1: Basic Balance
- Standing on One Leg: 3 sets of 10-30 seconds (each leg)
- Heel-to-Toe Walk: 3 sets of 10 steps
- Seated March: 3 sets of 10-15 lifts (each leg)

Day 2: Intermediate Balance
- Balance on an Unstable Surface: 3 sets of 10-30 seconds
- Single-Leg Deadlift: 3 sets of 10-15 reps (each leg)
- Side Leg Lift: 3 sets of 10-15 reps (each leg)

Day 3: Rest

Day 4: Advanced Balance
- Bosu Ball Squats: 3 sets of 10-15 reps

- Tandem Stand with Eyes Closed: 3 sets of 10-30 seconds
- Tai Chi: 20-30 minutes of practice

Day 5: Basic Balance
- Standing on One Leg: 3 sets of 10-30 seconds (each leg)
- Heel-to-Toe Walk: 3 sets of 10 steps
- Seated March: 3 sets of 10-15 lifts (each leg)

Day 6: Intermediate Balance
- Balance on an Unstable Surface: 3 sets of 10-30 seconds
- Single-Leg Deadlift: 3 sets of 10-15 reps (each leg)
- Side Leg Lift: 3 sets of 10-15 reps (each leg)

Day 7: Rest

Staying Motivated

Staying motivated can be challenging, especially during recovery. Here are some tips to keep you on track:

- Track Your Progress: Keep a journal or use an app to log your exercises and progress.
- Set Short-Term Goals: Break your long-term goals into smaller, achievable milestones.
- Find a Workout Buddy: Exercising with a friend can make workouts more enjoyable and keep you accountable.
- Celebrate Achievements: Reward yourself when you reach your goals, no matter how small.

Balance and coordination exercises are crucial components of injury recovery. They help improve stability, enhance coordination, strengthen muscles, boost confidence, and prevent future injuries. By consulting a healthcare provider, setting clear goals, starting with simple exercises, gradually increasing difficulty, focusing on proper form, and staying motivated, you can effectively use balance and coordination exercises to support your recovery. Remember, consistency and patience are key. With the right approach, you can regain your balance and coordination and get back to enjoying your favorite activities.

Chapter 15: Mental Health and Injury Recovery

Recovering from an injury isn't just about healing the body; it's also about taking care of your mind. Injuries can affect your mental health, leading to feelings of frustration, sadness, and anxiety. This chapter will explore why mental health is important during injury recovery, how to manage emotional challenges, and ways to stay positive and motivated. By the end, you'll understand how to take care of your mental health while healing your body.

Why Mental Health is Important
When you're injured, it's normal to feel down. Here are some reasons why mental health is crucial during recovery:

- Emotional Well-being: Injuries can lead to stress, sadness, and even depression. Taking care of your mental health can help you feel better emotionally.

- Motivation: Staying positive helps you stay motivated to stick with your rehabilitation plan.

- Pain Management: Stress and anxiety can make pain feel worse. Good mental health can help you manage pain better.

- Overall Recovery: A positive mindset can speed up the recovery process and help you heal more completely.

- Quality of Life: Good mental health improves your overall quality of life, making it easier to return to your daily activities and hobbies.

Understanding Emotional Challenges

Injury recovery can bring various emotional challenges. Understanding these challenges can help you address them effectively:

- Frustration: You may feel frustrated by your limited abilities or slow progress.
- Sadness: You might feel sad or down about missing out on activities you enjoy.
- Anxiety: Worries about your recovery and future health can cause anxiety.
- Isolation: Being unable to participate in social activities can make you feel lonely.
- Loss of Identity: If your injury prevents you from doing something you love, like a sport or hobby, you may feel a loss of identity.

Steps to Take Care of Your Mental Health

Taking care of your mental health during injury recovery is essential. Here are some steps to help you stay positive and motivated:

1. Acknowledge Your Feelings

It's okay to feel upset about your injury. Recognizing and accepting your emotions is the first step toward managing them. Don't ignore or suppress your feelings. Instead, talk about them with someone you trust, like a friend, family member, or therapist.

2. Stay Connected

Social support is crucial for mental health. Stay connected with friends and family, even if you can't participate in all activities. Here are some ways to stay connected:

- Phone Calls and Video Chats: Stay in touch with loved ones through phone calls or video chats.
- Social Media: Use social media to connect with friends and join support groups.
- Visits: Invite friends and family over for a visit.

3. Set Realistic Goals

Setting realistic goals can help you stay motivated and focused. Break your recovery into small, achievable steps. Celebrate each milestone, no matter how small, to keep your spirits high.

4. Stay Active

Physical activity can boost your mood and reduce stress. Even if you're limited in what you can do, find ways to stay active:

- Gentle Exercises: Try gentle exercises approved by your healthcare provider, like stretching or walking.
- Physical Therapy: Follow your physical therapy plan to stay active and promote healing.
- Mind-Body Activities: Activities like yoga or tai chi can help improve both physical and mental well-being.

5. Practice Relaxation Techniques

Relaxation techniques can help reduce stress and improve your mood. Here are some methods to try:

- Deep Breathing: Take slow, deep breaths to calm your mind and body.

- Meditation: Practice meditation to reduce stress and improve focus.
- Visualization: Imagine a peaceful place or positive outcome to help relax your mind.

6. Maintain a Routine

Keeping a daily routine can provide structure and a sense of normalcy. Here are some tips:

- Set a Schedule: Plan your day, including times for exercise, rest, and social activities.
- Stick to a Sleep Schedule: Go to bed and wake up at the same time each day to ensure good sleep.
- Include Enjoyable Activities: Make time for hobbies and activities you enjoy, even if you need to modify them.

7. Seek Professional Help

If you're struggling with your mental health, don't hesitate to seek professional help. A therapist or counselor can provide support and strategies to help you cope with your emotions. They can also help you address any anxiety, depression, or other mental health issues.

Staying Positive and Motivated

Staying positive and motivated during recovery can be challenging, but it's essential for your mental health. Here are some tips to help you stay upbeat:

- Focus on What You Can Do: Instead of dwelling on what you can't do, focus on the activities you can still enjoy.
- Stay Informed: Learn about your injury and recovery process. Knowledge can reduce anxiety and help you feel more in control.
- Use Positive Self-Talk: Encourage yourself with positive thoughts and affirmations.
- Find Inspiration: Read stories or watch videos about others who have successfully recovered from injuries.

- Reward Yourself: Celebrate your progress with small rewards, like a favorite treat or activity.

Mental health is a vital part of injury recovery. By acknowledging your feelings, staying connected, setting realistic goals, staying active, practicing relaxation techniques, maintaining a routine, and seeking professional help when needed, you can take care of your mental health while healing your body. Staying positive and motivated will help you overcome emotional challenges and speed up your recovery. Remember, you're not alone, and with the right approach, you can come out stronger and healthier, both physically and mentally.

Chapter 16: Preventing Re-Injury

After working hard to recover from an injury, the last thing you want is to get hurt again. Preventing re-injury is crucial to ensure you can enjoy your favorite activities without setbacks. This chapter will explain why preventing re-injury is important, share practical tips to stay safe, and guide you through creating a plan to protect yourself. By the end, you'll have the knowledge to keep your body strong and healthy, reducing the risk of getting injured again.

Why Preventing Re-Injury is Important

Re-injury can be frustrating and discouraging. Here are some reasons why it's important to prevent it:

- Maintain Progress: Avoiding re-injury helps you maintain the progress you've made in your recovery.
- Reduce Pain: Re-injury can lead to more pain and longer recovery times.
- Boost Confidence: Staying injury-free boosts your confidence in your ability to return to normal activities.
- Save Time and Money: Preventing re-injury saves you from spending more time and money on medical treatments and therapy.
- Enhance Quality of Life: Staying healthy allows you to participate in activities you love, improving your overall quality of life.

Understanding Risk Factors

Understanding what can increase your risk of re-injury helps you take proactive steps to stay safe. Here are some common risk factors:

- Returning Too Soon: Going back to activities before you're fully healed can increase the risk of re-injury.
- Poor Technique: Using improper techniques in sports or daily activities can strain your body.
- Lack of Strength and Flexibility: Weak muscles and lack of flexibility make you more prone to injuries.
- Overtraining: Pushing your body too hard without adequate rest can lead to overuse injuries.
- Ignoring Pain: Ignoring pain and continuing activities can worsen injuries.

Steps to Prevent Re-Injury

Preventing re-injury involves a combination of proper training, good habits, and listening to your body. Follow these steps to stay safe and healthy:

1. Follow Your Rehabilitation Plan

Sticking to your rehabilitation plan is crucial for full recovery. Here's how to do it:

- Complete All Exercises: Perform all the exercises recommended by your physical therapist or doctor.
- Attend Follow-Up Appointments: Regularly check in with your healthcare provider to monitor your progress.
- Be Patient: Healing takes time. Don't rush the process.

2. Use Proper Technique

Using the correct technique in sports and daily activities reduces the risk of injury. Here are some tips:

- Learn from Experts: Take lessons or seek guidance from coaches and trainers to learn proper techniques.
- Practice Good Form: Focus on maintaining good form during exercises and activities.
- Adjust Movements: Modify your movements if you experience pain or discomfort.

3. Strengthen Muscles

Strong muscles support your joints and reduce the risk of injury. Here are some ways to build strength:

- Strength Training: Incorporate strength training exercises into your routine to target key muscle groups.
- Core Exercises: Strengthen your core muscles, as they play a vital role in overall stability.
- Balanced Workouts: Ensure your workouts include exercises for all major muscle groups to avoid imbalances.

4. Improve Flexibility

Flexible muscles and joints are less likely to get injured. Here's how to improve flexibility:

- Stretch Regularly: Incorporate stretching into your daily routine to maintain flexibility.

- Warm-Up and Cool Down: Always warm up before exercises and cool down afterward with gentle stretches.
- Yoga or Pilates: Try yoga or Pilates to improve flexibility and balance.

5. Listen to Your Body

Paying attention to your body's signals helps prevent overuse and strain. Here's what to do:

- Recognize Pain: Stop activities if you feel pain. Pain is a sign that something may be wrong.
- Rest When Needed: Take breaks and allow your body to rest and recover.
- Adjust Activities: Modify or avoid activities that cause discomfort or pain.

6. Gradually Increase Activity

Increasing your activity level gradually helps prevent re-injury. Here's how to do it:

- Start Slow: Begin with low-intensity activities and gradually increase the intensity and duration.
- Set Realistic Goals: Set achievable goals for your return to activities and progress slowly.
- Monitor Progress: Keep track of your progress and make adjustments as needed.

7. Use Proper Equipment

Using the right equipment and gear can protect you from injuries. Here are some tips:

- Wear Appropriate Shoes: Choose shoes that provide good support and fit well for your activities.
- Use Protective Gear: Wear protective gear like helmets, knee pads, or braces when needed.
- Maintain Equipment: Regularly check and maintain your equipment to ensure it's in good condition.

Creating a Re-Injury Prevention Plan

Having a plan in place helps you stay on track and reduce the risk of re-injury. Here's how to create one:

1. Set Clear Goals
Setting clear, specific goals helps you stay focused. Here are some examples:

- Strength Goal: "I will perform strength training exercises three times a week to build muscle."
- Flexibility Goal: "I will stretch for 10 minutes each day to improve my flexibility."
- Technique Goal: "I will take a weekly class to learn proper techniques for my sport."

2. Develop a Routine
A consistent routine helps you stay committed to your prevention plan. Here's how to do it:

- Schedule Workouts: Plan your workouts and stick to a regular schedule.

- Include Variety: Incorporate different types of exercises to keep your routine balanced and interesting.
- Track Progress: Use a journal or app to log your activities and monitor your progress.

3. Seek Support

Having support from others can keep you motivated and accountable. Here are some ideas:

- Workout Buddy: Find a friend or family member to exercise with and share your goals.
- Professional Guidance: Work with a trainer, coach, or physical therapist to stay on track.
- Join a Community: Join a fitness group or online community for support and encouragement.

Preventing re-injury is essential for maintaining your progress, reducing pain, boosting confidence, saving time and money, and enhancing your quality of life. By following your rehabilitation plan, using proper technique, strengthening muscles, improving flexibility, listening to your body, gradually increasing activity, and using proper equipment, you can protect yourself from getting injured again. Creating a re-injury prevention plan with clear goals, a consistent routine, and support from others will help you stay on track. Remember, taking care of your body is a lifelong commitment. With the right approach, you can stay healthy and enjoy your favorite activities without setbacks.

Chapter 17: Adapting Daily Activities

Recovering from an injury often means you need to adjust how you go about your daily activities. These changes can help you heal faster and prevent further injuries. This chapter will guide you through understanding why adapting your daily activities is important, practical tips for making these changes, and how to stay positive and motivated throughout the process. By the end, you'll know how to make your daily routine safer and more comfortable as you recover.

Why Adapting Daily Activities is Important

Making adjustments to your daily activities is crucial for several reasons:

- Promote Healing: Giving your injured body part the rest it needs helps speed up recovery.
- Prevent Further Injury: Proper adaptations can help you avoid movements that might worsen your injury.
- Manage Pain: Modifying activities can reduce pain and discomfort.
- Maintain Independence: Adapting your activities allows you to stay independent and continue with your routine as much as possible.
- Boost Confidence: Successfully managing your daily tasks despite your injury can boost your confidence and mood.

Understanding the Challenges

Adapting to new ways of doing things can be challenging. Here are some common difficulties you might face:

- Frustration: It's normal to feel frustrated when you can't do things the way you used to.

- Fear of Making It Worse: You might worry about doing something that could aggravate your injury.
- Learning New Techniques: It can take time to learn and get used to new methods for everyday tasks.
- Physical Limitations: Pain or limited movement can make certain activities harder to perform.
- Emotional Impact: Feeling dependent or limited can affect your mood and self-esteem.

Steps to Adapt Your Daily Activities

Adjusting your daily routine doesn't have to be overwhelming. Here are some steps to help you adapt effectively:

1. Identify Activities That Need Adjustment

Start by identifying which activities are affected by your injury. This could include tasks like:

- Getting Dressed: Buttoning shirts or tying shoelaces might be challenging.

- Cooking and Eating: Preparing food and handling utensils might be difficult.
- Cleaning and Chores: Tasks like vacuuming, lifting laundry, or washing dishes may need to be modified.
- Work and Hobbies: Typing, writing, or engaging in physical hobbies could be impacted.

2. Use Assistive Devices

Assistive devices can make many tasks easier and safer. Here are some examples:

- Reachers and Grabbers: Help you pick up items without bending or stretching.
- Shower Chairs and Grab Bars: Make bathing safer and more comfortable.
- Adaptive Utensils: Specially designed tools for eating, cooking, and other tasks.
- Braces and Supports: Provide stability and reduce strain on the injured area.

3. Modify Your Environment

Changing your environment can help you perform tasks more easily. Consider these modifications:

- Rearrange Furniture: Create clear pathways and make frequently used items easily accessible.
- Adjust Workspaces: Modify your desk setup to reduce strain, such as using an ergonomic chair or keyboard.
- Use Proper Lighting: Ensure good lighting to avoid unnecessary strain and accidents.
- Organize Closets and Cabinets: Place frequently used items at waist height to avoid bending or stretching.

4. Break Tasks into Smaller Steps

Breaking tasks into smaller, manageable steps can make them less overwhelming. Here's how:

- Plan Ahead: Organize your day and prioritize tasks to avoid overexertion.

- Take Breaks: Give yourself permission to take breaks and rest as needed.
- Do One Thing at a Time: Focus on completing one task before moving on to the next.

5. Ask for Help

Don't hesitate to ask for help when you need it. Here are some ways to get support:

- Family and Friends: Ask loved ones to assist with tasks that are difficult or painful.
- Professional Services: Consider hiring help for tasks like cleaning, shopping, or yard work.
- Support Groups: Join a support group for people with similar injuries for advice and encouragement.

6. Practice Good Body Mechanics

Using proper body mechanics can help prevent further injury and make tasks easier. Here are some tips:

- Lift with Your Legs: Bend at your knees, not your back, when lifting objects.
- Keep Items Close: Hold objects close to your body to reduce strain.
- Avoid Twisting: Turn your whole body instead of twisting at the waist.
- Use Both Hands: Distribute the weight of objects evenly between both hands.

7. Stay Positive and Patient

Adapting to new ways of doing things takes time and patience. Here are some tips to stay positive:

- Celebrate Small Wins: Acknowledge and celebrate your progress, no matter how small.
- Stay Focused on Your Goals: Remind yourself of the bigger picture and your recovery goals.
- Be Kind to Yourself: Understand that it's okay to have bad days and setbacks.

- Find Joy in New Ways: Discover new activities and hobbies that you can enjoy within your current limitations.

Adapting your daily activities is essential for promoting healing, preventing further injury, managing pain, maintaining independence, and boosting confidence. By identifying activities that need adjustment, using assistive devices, modifying your environment, breaking tasks into smaller steps, asking for help, practicing good body mechanics, and staying positive and patient, you can make your daily routine safer and more comfortable. Remember, recovery is a journey, and making these changes will help you get back to doing the things you love more quickly and safely.

Chapter 18: Long-Term Recovery Strategies

Recovering from an injury is a journey that doesn't end when the pain goes away or when you finish physical therapy. Long-term recovery is about staying healthy and strong, so you don't get hurt again and can enjoy your favorite activities. This chapter will help you understand why long-term recovery is important, give you practical tips, and show you how to keep these strategies in your daily life. By the end, you'll know how to support your body and stay healthy for the long run.

Why Long-Term Recovery is Important

Sticking to a long-term recovery plan is important for several reasons:

- Keep Your Progress: Ensure that all the hard work you've put into healing doesn't go to waste.
- Avoid Future Injuries: Strengthen your body to reduce the risk of getting hurt again.
- Stay Healthy: Promote overall well-being and fitness through good habits.
- Enjoy Life: Participate in activities you love without setbacks.
- Build Confidence: Trust in your body's ability to handle daily tasks and physical activities.

Challenges You Might Face

Long-term recovery has its challenges. Here are some you might encounter:

- Staying Consistent: Keeping up with your recovery plan over time.
- Maintaining Motivation: Finding the drive to continue exercises and healthy habits.
- Time Management: Balancing recovery activities with a busy schedule.

- Hitting Plateaus: Experiencing times when progress seems slow or stops.
- Physical Limits: Dealing with any lingering limitations or chronic pain.

Steps for Long-Term Recovery

Here are some steps to help you maintain your progress and support your body over time:

1. Keep Doing Your Physical Therapy Exercises

Continue the exercises you learned in physical therapy. Here's how to stay on track:

- Make a Routine: Schedule your exercises into your daily or weekly routine.
- Mix Things Up: Add variety to your exercises to keep them interesting and target different muscles.
- Stay Dedicated: Remember that these exercises are essential for maintaining your recovery.

2. Stay Active

Regular physical activity is crucial for long-term recovery. Here's how to keep moving:

- Find Fun Activities: Choose activities you enjoy, like walking, swimming, or biking.
- Set Goals: Create fitness goals to keep yourself motivated.
- Join a Group: Participate in fitness classes or group activities for accountability and social support.

3. Strengthen Your Core

A strong core supports your whole body and helps prevent injuries. Here's how to focus on your core:

- Core Exercises: Do exercises like planks, bridges, and abdominal workouts.
- Try Yoga or Pilates: These activities are great for building core strength and flexibility.
- Be Consistent: Include core workouts in your regular exercise routine.

4. Stay Flexible

Keeping your muscles and joints flexible helps prevent injuries. Here's how to stay flexible:

- Stretch Daily: Make stretching a part of your daily routine.
- Warm Up and Cool Down: Always warm up before and cool down after physical activities.
- Stay Active: Regular physical activity helps maintain flexibility.

5. Track Your Progress

Keeping track of your progress helps you stay motivated and make necessary adjustments. Here's what to do:

- Write It Down: Use a journal or an app to record your exercises, activities, and any changes in how you feel.

- Set Milestones: Create milestones to celebrate your progress and stay motivated.
- Adjust When Needed: If you hit a plateau or feel pain, adjust your routine and consult a healthcare professional.

6. Listen to Your Body

Pay attention to your body's signals to avoid overuse and injury. Here's how to listen to your body:

- Recognize Pain: If something hurts, stop and rest. Don't push through pain.
- Rest When Needed: Give yourself time to recover, especially after intense activities.
- Stay Educated: Learn about your body and what it needs to stay healthy.

7. Practice Healthy Habits

Healthy habits support your body's recovery and overall well-being. Here are some to consider:

- Eat a Balanced Diet: Consume a diet rich in nutrients to support muscle recovery and overall health.
- Stay Hydrated: Drink plenty of water to stay hydrated and support bodily functions.
- Get Enough Sleep: Ensure you get enough sleep to allow your body to repair and recover.

8. Stay Positive and Motivated

Maintaining a positive attitude and motivation is key to long-term recovery. Here are some tips:

- Set Realistic Goals: Set achievable goals to keep yourself motivated.
- Celebrate Small Wins: Acknowledge and celebrate your progress, no matter how small.
- Stay Connected: Engage with friends, family, or support groups for motivation and encouragement.

Long-term recovery strategies are essential for keeping your progress, avoiding future injuries, staying healthy, enjoying life, and building confidence. By continuing physical therapy exercises, staying active, strengthening your core, maintaining flexibility, tracking your progress, listening to your body, practicing healthy habits, and staying positive and motivated, you can support your body for the long haul. Remember, recovery is a continuous journey, and maintaining these strategies will help you stay strong, healthy, and injury-free.

Chapter 19: Success Stories and Case Studies

Hearing about other people's experiences can be incredibly motivating and helpful when you're on your recovery journey. In this chapter, we will share success stories and case studies of individuals who have faced injuries and come out stronger on the other side. These real-life examples will show you that with dedication, perseverance, and the right strategies, you can overcome challenges and achieve a successful recovery. By the end, you'll be inspired by their journeys and have valuable insights to apply to your own recovery.

Jennifer's Journey: Overcoming a Knee Injury
Emily loved skiing, but one winter, she had a serious knee injury. It was painful, and she was

worried she might never ski again. But Emily was determined to get better. Here's how she did it:

- Physical Therapy: Emily started with physical therapy, focusing on exercises to strengthen her knee and regain mobility.
- Consistency: She made a habit of doing her exercises every day, even when she didn't feel like it.
- Staying Active: Once her knee was stronger, Emily took up yoga to improve her flexibility and balance.
- Gradual Return to Skiing: She slowly reintroduced skiing, starting with easy slopes and gradually taking on more challenging ones.
- Support System: Emily leaned on her friends and family for support and encouragement.

Today, Emily is back on the slopes, enjoying skiing more than ever. Her journey shows that with patience and hard work, you can return to doing what you love.

Carlos's Recovery: From Shoulder Injury to Strength

Carlos was an avid weightlifter, but he suffered a shoulder injury that put his passion on hold. The road to recovery was tough, but Carlos managed to come back even stronger. Here's his story:

- Initial Setback: After injuring his shoulder, Carlos had to stop lifting weights and focus on healing.
- Rehabilitation Exercises: He worked closely with a physical therapist to do specific exercises that targeted his shoulder muscles.
- Focus on Core Strength: Carlos also worked on strengthening his core to support his overall fitness.
- Adjusting Workouts: He modified his workout routine to include exercises that didn't strain his shoulder.
- Mindset: Carlos kept a positive attitude, setting small, achievable goals and celebrating each milestone.

Now, Carlos is lifting weights again, but he's smarter about his workouts. He learned the importance of proper form and listening to his body, which has made him a better athlete.

Sarah's Transformation: Healing a Chronic Back Issue

Sarah struggled with chronic back pain for years, affecting her daily life and making it hard to enjoy her favorite activities. Here's how she turned things around:

- Seeking Help: Sarah consulted with doctors and physical therapists to understand her back pain.
- Customized Exercise Plan: She followed a personalized exercise plan that focused on strengthening her back and core muscles.
- Lifestyle Changes: Sarah made changes to her lifestyle, like improving her posture and setting up an ergonomic workspace.

- Mindfulness and Relaxation: She practiced mindfulness and relaxation techniques to manage stress and reduce muscle tension.
- Perseverance: Sarah was committed to her recovery plan, even on tough days.

Today, Sarah's back pain is under control, and she enjoys hiking and yoga. Her story shows that with the right approach and persistence, you can overcome chronic pain.

John's Comeback: Managing a Sports Injury

John was a passionate basketball player until he injured his ankle. He was afraid he might never play again, but he didn't give up. Here's how John made his comeback:

- Rest and Recovery: John started with plenty of rest to allow his ankle to heal properly.

- Rehabilitation: He followed a structured rehabilitation program to regain strength and mobility in his ankle.

- Gradual Return: John gradually reintroduced basketball drills, starting with light exercises and progressing to more intense ones.

- Support Network: He relied on his teammates, coach, and family for support and motivation.

- Ongoing Maintenance: John continues to do exercises to keep his ankle strong and prevent future injuries.

Now, John is back on the basketball court, playing with the same passion and energy as before his injury. His story is a testament to the power of determination and a well-structured recovery plan.

Anna's Success: Overcoming a Hip Injury

Anna loved running marathons, but a hip injury forced her to stop. She feared she might never run again, but she was determined to recover. Here's how Anna did it:

- Medical Consultation: Anna worked with doctors to understand her injury and the best way to heal.
- Physical Therapy: She diligently followed her physical therapy routine to strengthen her hip and improve flexibility.
- Cross-Training: Anna took up swimming and cycling to stay active without putting stress on her hip.
- Patience: She gave herself time to heal, avoiding rushing back into running.
- Gradual Progress: Anna gradually reintroduced running, starting with short distances and slowly increasing.

Today, Anna is back to running marathons, enjoying the sport she loves. Her journey shows that patience and a well-rounded approach to recovery can lead to a successful comeback.

Lessons Learned from Success Stories

These success stories highlight several key lessons:

- Consistency is Key: Regular exercise and following a recovery plan are crucial for long-term success.
- Stay Positive: A positive attitude and setting small, achievable goals can keep you motivated.
- Seek Support: Rely on friends, family, and professionals for encouragement and guidance.
- Listen to Your Body: Pay attention to your body's signals and avoid pushing through pain.
- Be Patient: Recovery takes time, so be patient and give yourself the time you need to heal.

Conclusion

Recovering from an injury is a journey filled with ups and downs, but it is a journey worth taking. Throughout this book, we've explored the various aspects of injury recovery, from understanding common injuries and the phases of healing to the importance of physical therapy, setting realistic goals, and maintaining long-term recovery strategies.

Injury recovery is not just about physical healing. It's about rebuilding your strength, regaining your confidence, and learning to listen to your body. It involves a holistic approach, incorporating physical exercises, proper nutrition, mental health support, and lifestyle adjustments.

Key Takeaways

1. Immediate Response is Crucial: Knowing how to respond immediately after an injury can significantly impact your recovery process. Proper care right from the start sets a strong foundation for healing.

2. Role of Medical Professionals: Seeking advice and treatment from medical professionals ensures you get the right diagnosis and tailored recovery plan. They are your partners in this journey, providing guidance and support.

3. Setting Realistic Goals: Setting achievable recovery goals keeps you motivated and focused. Celebrate small milestones along the way; they are signs of progress.

4. Importance of Rest and Recovery: Allowing your body time to rest and recover is as important as the exercises you do. It helps prevent overuse injuries and promotes overall healing.

5. Nutrition and Pain Management: Eating a balanced diet and using effective pain management techniques support your body's healing process and enhance your comfort.

6. Benefits of Physical Therapy: Physical therapy plays a vital role in rehabilitation. It helps restore function, improve mobility, and prevent future injuries.

7. Creating a Rehabilitation Plan: A structured rehabilitation plan is your roadmap to recovery. Stick to it, but be flexible and adjust as needed based on your progress and how your body feels.

8. Exercise and Fitness: Incorporating stretching, flexibility exercises, strength training, cardiovascular conditioning, and balance exercises into your routine supports your overall recovery and prevents re-injury.

9. Mental Health: Taking care of your mental health is crucial during recovery. Stay positive, seek support, and practice stress-relief techniques to maintain a healthy mind and body.

10. Long-Term Strategies: Long-term recovery strategies ensure that you maintain the progress you've made. Stay active, continue your exercises, and integrate healthy habits into your daily life.

Moving Forward

Remember, recovery is a continuous journey. The success stories and case studies we've shared show that with determination, the right strategies, and a supportive network, you can overcome injuries and achieve a full recovery. Each person's journey is unique, and it's essential to find what works best for you.

Stay committed to your recovery plan, listen to your body, and don't be afraid to seek help when needed. Celebrate your progress, no matter how small, and stay motivated by setting new goals.

Injury recovery is not just about getting back to where you were before the injury; it's about becoming stronger, wiser, and more resilient. Embrace this journey with an open mind and a positive attitude. You have
the tools and knowledge to support your body and mind, ensuring a healthy and active life ahead.

www.ingramcontent.com/pod-product-compliance
Lightning Source LLC
Chambersburg PA
CBHW071921210526
45479CB00002B/500